1. _____ Is an example of a patient protection technique used before x-ray exposure.
   a. Proper film processing
   b. Proper prescribing of radiographs
   c. A lead apron
   d. A thyroid collar

2. The Collimator:
   a. Is always round
   b. Restricts the size and shape of the x-ray beam
   c. Is a solid piece of aluminum

3. Which Type of PID would be most effective in reducing patient exposure?
   a. Conical
   b. 16 inch round PID
   c. 8 inch rectangular PID
   d. 16-inch rectangular PID

4. Speed film is currently the fastest intraoral film available?
   a. D
   b. E
   c. F
   d. G

5. On some dental x-ray machines, only the ___ can be altered; the other parameters are preset by the manufacturer.
   a. Kilovoltage peak
   b. Exposure Time
   c. PID length
   d. Milliamperage

6. Which one occurrences during and after x-ray film exposure reduce(s) the amount of x-radiation a patient receives?
   a. Artifacts caused by improper film handling
   b. Retakes
   c. Proper film processing
   d. Nondiagnostic films

7. According to the current recommendations (2003) of the National Council on Radiation Protection and Measurements, The Current MPD for an occupationally exposed pregnant woman is the same as that for:
a. An occupationally exposed nonpregnant women
b. An occupationally exposed male
c. An occupationally exposed child under 18
d. A non occupationally exposed person

8. The Acronym for the permitted lifetime accumulated dose is:
a. MPD- Maximum permissible dose
b. MPD-Maximum possible dose
c. MAD-Maximum accumulated dose
d. MAD-Maximum allowed dose

9. The ___allow(s) for positioning of the tubehead
a. Control devices
b. Extension arm
c. Control Panel
d. Exposure Button

10. The ___activate(s) The machine to produce x-rays.
a. on/off switch
b. Exposure button
c. Exposure light
d. Control devices

11. Which of the following intraoral film holders is a disposable Styrofoam bite block?
a. EEZEE-Grip
b. Stabe bite block
c. EndoRay
d. Uni-bite

12. The Film emulsion is:
a. Attached to both sides of the film
b. Attached to one side of the film
c. Made of polyester plastic
d. Opaque to block out the passage of light

13. The label side of the dental film packet:
a. Is solid white
b. Has a raised bump in one corner that corresponds to the identification dot
c. Should face the tubehead when placed in the mouth
d. Is colored coded to distinguish between one film and two film packets and between film speeds

14. Which of the following types of film exhibits the bony and soft tissue areas of the facial profile?
a. Periapical
b. Bitewing
c. Panoramic
d. Cephalometric

15. Film is best stored in an area that is :
    a. Hot
    b. Humid
    c. Cool and dry
    d. Exposed to radiation

16. Which of the following areas would appear the most radiolucent on a Dental Radiograph?
a. Composite
b. Amalgam
c. Air space
d. Enamel

17. Radiolucent refers to that portion of a processed radiograph that is:
a. Black
b. White
c. Gray
d. Coated with emulsion

18. Radiopaque refers to that portion of a processed radiograph that is:
a. Black
b. White
c. Gray
d. Within the plastic base

19. Which of the following changes will result in a radiograph with reduced density?
    a. Increasing the exposure time
    b. Increasing the subject thickness
    c. Increasing the milliamperage
    d. Increasing the operating kilovoltage peak

20. A step wedge will reveal that radiographs taken at a higher KVp will have __Versus radiographs taken at a lower kVp.
    a. Long scale contrast
    b. High contrast
    c. Only two densities
    d. Many areas of black and white

21. The primary factor that limits the size of the tungsten target is:
    a. The cost of the materials
    b. Heat production
    c. The limited kinetic energy of the electrons
    d. The limited Kinetic energy of the protons

22. During processing, a chemical reaction occurs, and the halide portion of the __ silver halide crystal is removed.
    a. Unexposed, Unergized
    b. Exposed, unenergized
    c. Unexposed, energized
    d. Exposed, energized

23. Which type of silver halide crystal are removed from the film?
    a. Unexposed, unergized
    b. Exposed, Unergized
    c. Unexposed, energized
    d. Exposed, energized

24. The purpose of ____ is to chemically reduce the exposed, energized silver halide crystal into black metallic silver.
   a. Developer
   b. Fixer
   c. Rinsing
   d. Washing

25. Normal use of processing chemistry is defined as ___ intraoral films per day.
   a. 18
   b. 30
   c. 50
   d. 60

26. ___ generates the black tones and the sharp contrast of the radiographic image.
   a. Sodium Sulfite
   b. Sodium Carbonate
   c. Hydroquinone
   d. Potassium Bromide

27. The preservative used in developer solution is:
   a. Hydroquinone
   b. Sodium sulfite
   c. Sodium carbonate
   d. Potassium bromide

28. The preservative used in developer solution is:
   a. Silver halide
   b. Silver bromide
   c. Air
   d. Moisture

29. Which of the following chemicals is the accelerator in developer solution?
   a. Hydroquinone
   b. Elon
   c. Sodium Sulfite
   d. Sodium Carbonate

30. The restrainer stops the development of:
   a. Unexposed crystals only
   b. Exposed crystals only
   c. Unexposed crystals more than exposed crystals
   d. Exposed crystals more than unexposed crystals

31. Which of the following is a component of fixer solution, but not developer solution?
   a. Potassium bromide
   b. Potassium alum
   c. Hydroquinone
   d. Sodium Carbonate

32. Sodium sulfite is the ___used in fixer solution.
   a. Fixing
   b. Preservative
   c. Hardening Agent
   d. Acidifier

33. The purpose of the hardening agent is to harden and shrink the:
   a. Exposed silver halide crystals
   b. Unexposed silver halide crystals
   c. Gelatin in the film emulsion
   d. Plastic Film Base

34. The master tank is filled with:
   a. Developer
   b. Fixer
   c. Cold Water
   d. Temperature-controlled water

35. The temperatures of the developer and fixer solutions are controlled by the:
   a. Ambient room temperature
   b. Aquarium-type heaters in the insert tanks
   c. Use of mixing valve
   d. Chemical reaction that occurs when they are mixed

36. A thermometer may be clipped to the side of the ___ for manual processing.
    a. Developer tank
    b. Fixer tank
    c. Master tank
    d. Both insert tanks

37. Developer solution should be changed ___ fixer solution.
    a. Twice as often as
    b. More often than
    c. Less often than
    d. At the same time as

38. Deposits form on the inside walls of insert tanks because of an interaction between mineral salts in water ___ process solutions.
    a. Sodium thiosulfate
    b. Carbonate
    c. Acetic acid
    d. Hydroquinone

39. Which of the following would be the best choice for cleaning the master and insert tanks?
    a. Plain tap water
    b. A solution of hydrochloric acid and water
    c. A powder type abrasive cleanser
    d. A liquid type abrasive cleanser

40. The major advantage of automatic film processing versus manual film processing is:
    a. Less processing time is required.
    b. Time is manually controlled
    c. Water temperature is manually controlled
    d. More sophisticated equipment is used.

41. To conduct a film-screen contact test, the wire mesh test object is placed:
    a. On top of the loaded cassette
    b. On the side of the film closest to the tubehead within the loaded cassette
    c. On the side of the film farthest from the tubehead within the loaded cassette
    d. Over the end of the PID

42. The clearing test is used to monitor:
   a. Developer strength
   b. Fixer Strength
   c. Water bath temperature
   d. Processing speed

43. If the film clears in __minutes, the chemistry is of adequate strength.
   a. 2
   b. 6
   c. 8
   d. 14

44. The dental radiographer requires which of the following to perform dental radiographic procedures?
   a. Sufficient knowledge
   b. Technical skills
   c. Sufficient knowledge and technical skills
   d. Neither sufficient knowledge and technical skills

45. An oral examination limits the practitioner to knowledge of what is seen clinically. Dental x-rays allow the practitioner to see many conditions that are not apparent clinically.
   a. Both statements are true.
   b. Both statements are false
   c. The first statement is true; the second is false
   d. The first statement is false; the second is true

46. Radiographs enable the dental professional to see__conditions that may otherwise go undetected.
   a. Rare
   b. Occasional common
   c. Occasional
   d. Many

47. The consumer-Patient Radiation Health and Safety Act:Outlines requirements for the safe use of dental x-ray equipment.

1. Outlines requirements for the safe use of dental x-ray equipment.
2. Establishes guidelines for the proper maintenance of x-ray equipment.
3. Requires persons who take dental radiographs to be properly trained and certified.
   a. 1,2,3
   b. 1,2
   c. 2,3
   d. 1,3

48. Informed Consent:
   a. Must be in language that the patient can readily understand
   b. Does not require that patients have their questions answered before x-ray exposure
   c. Is waived if the patient is a minor
   d. Does not require that patients receive enough information to make informed choices

49. Which of the following statements is true of radiographs and the patient's dental record?
   a. Radiographs may be discarded when outdated
   b. It is advised to keep patient radiographs in a file separate from patients charts
   c. The dental record must include documentation of the number and type of radiographs exposed.
   d. Dental radiographs are an optional rather than an integral part of the dental record.

50. ____ is defined as the absence of pathogens, or disease causing microorganisms.
   a. Antiseptic
   b. Antibiotic
   c. Antinfective
   d. Asepsis

51. Antiseptic is:
   a. The absence of pathogens, or disease-causing microorganisms
   b. A substance that inhibits the growth of bacteria
   c. The use of a chemical or physical procedure to inhibit ordstroy pathogens
   d. The act of sterilizing

52. ___when using medical latex or vinyl gloves.
    a. Gloves may be rewashed between patients and reused until damaged.
    b. Non Sterile gloves are recommended for examinations and nonsurgical procedures.
    c. Hands should not be washed before gloving
    d. Hands should not be washed between patients.

53. Which of the following are considered to be semi critical instruments?
    a. The exposure button
    b. The x ray control panel
    c. The lead apron
    d. X ray film holding devices

54. Covering exposed surfaces with disposable materials ___adequate protection ___the need for surface cleaning and disinfection between patients.
    a. Provides; while eliminating
    b. Provides; but does not eliminate
    c. Does not provide; but does eliminate
    d. Neither provides; nor eliminates

55. Which of the following surfaces on the x-ray machine must be covered or disinfected?
    1. Control panel
    2. Exposure button
    3. Tubehead
    4. Position indicating devices (PID)
        a. 1,2,3,4
        b. 1,2,3
        c. 2,3,4
        d. 2 only

56. After seating the patient, the radiographer must complete which of the following procedures before washing the hands and putting on gloves?
   1. Chair adjustment
   2. Headrest adjustment
   3. Placing the lead apron

      a. 1,2,3
      b. 1,2
      c. 2,3
      d. 3 Only

57. When handling film with barrier envelopes, the films are unwrapped with___hands, and when handling film without barrier envelopes, The films are unwrapped with ___hands.
   a. Gloved, gloved
   b. Gloved non gloved
   c. Nongloved, gloved
   d. Nongloved, nongloved

58. There are___methods for obtaining Periapical radiographs.
   a. Two
   b. Three
   c. Five
   d. Ten

59. The CMRS is defined as a series of intraoral dental radiographs that shows:
   a. All the dentulous tooth-bearing areas of the upper and lower jaws
   b. All the endentulous tooth-bearing areas of the upper and lower jaws
   c. All the dentulous or edentulous tooth bearing areas of the upper and lower jaws.

60. When tori are present:
   a. The patient will require a panoramic film.
   b. The film should be placed on the torus and exposed.
   c. The patient should be referred for surgical tori reduction before films are taken.
   d. The film must be placed on the far side of the torus.

61. All crowns and roots of the first, second, and third molars, including the apices, alveolar crest, contact areas, surrounding bone, and tuberosity region, must be seen on the ___radiograph.
    a. Maxillary premolar
    b. Maxillary molar
    c. Mandibular premolar
    d. Mandibular molar

62. The primary benefit of using film holders with the bisecting technique is:
    a. Assisting in determining vertical angulation
    b. Helping to minimize cone cuts
    c. Reducing the patient's exposure to radiation
    d. Allowing the operator to have the film parallel to the long axis of the tooth

63. Which of the following commercially available film holders can be used with the bisecting technique?
    a. Rinn BAI instruments
    b. Rinn XCP instruments
    c. Stabe bite block
    d. Both a and c

64. With the finger holding method, which of the following would be used to hold the maxillary right molar film?
    a. Left thumb
    b. Right thumb
    c. Left finger
    d. Right finger

65. Elongated images refer to images of the teeth that appear ___, Elongation of the images results from ___vertical angulation.
    a. Too long; excessive
    b. To long; insufficient
    c. Shortened; excessive
    d. Shortened; insufficient

66. With size 2 film, a total of ___ anterior film placements are used in the bisecting technique.
    a. Four
    b. Six
    c. Seven
    d. Eight

67. The primary disadvantage of the bisecting technique when contrasted with the paralleling technique is:
    a. Longer exposure times
    b. Dimensional distortion
    c. Requirement of a film holder
    d. Greater magnification

68. For the maxillary premolar exposure, the front edge of the film should be aligned with the midline of the maxillary:
    a. Lateral incisor
    b. Canine
    c. First premolar
    d. Second premolar

69. With the bisecting technique, the recommended vertical angulation range for maxillary canines is ___ degrees.
    a. +20 to +30
    b. +30 to +40
    c. +40 to +50
    d. +45 to +55

70. The bite-wing tab is a heavy paperboard tab or loop fitted around a periapical film and used to stabilize the film during exposure. The periapical film is oriented in the bite loop so that the tab portion extends from the white side(tube side) of the film.
    a. Both statements are true
    b. Both statements are false
    c. The first statement is true; the second statement is false.
    d. The first statement is false; the second statement is true.

71. ____sizes of bite-wing films are available.
    a. Two
    b. Three
    c. Four
    d. Six

72. Which size of bite- wing film is used to examine the posterior teeth of children with mixed dentition?
    a. Size 0
    b. Size 1
    c. Size 2
    d. Size 3

73. In the adult patient, which size film is recommended for bite-wing exposures?
    a. Size 0
    b. Size 1
    c. Size 2
    d. Size 3

74. The problem with a single bite-wing film per side for adult patients is increased:
    a. X-ray exposure
    b. Possibility of inciting the gag reflex
    c. Overlapped contacts
    d. Useful diagnostic information

75. When determining vertical angulation, if the position-indicating device (PID) is positioned above the occlusal plane and the central ray is directed_ , the vertical angulation is termed____.
    a. Upward; positive
    b. Downward;positive
    c. Upward; negative
    d. downward ; negative

76. For the premolar bite-wing exposure, the PID is positioned far enough forward to cover both maxillary and mandibular.
    a. Lateral incisors
    b. Canines
    c. First premolars
    d. Second Premolars

77. For the premolar bite-wing exposure, the PID is positioned far enough forward to cover both maxillary and mandibular.
    a. Lateral incisors
    b. Canines
    c. First premolars
    d. Second premolars

78. For the molar bite-wing exposure, the front edge of the film should be aligned with the midline of the :
    a. Maxillary first premolar
    b. Mandibular first premolar
    c. Maxillary second premolar
    d. Mandibular second premolar

79. An unexposed film appears:
    a. Clear
    b. Black
    c. Dark
    d. Light

80. When the occlusal plane appears tipped or tilted, the error is a (n):
    a. Incorrect horizontal angulation
    b. Incorrect vertical angulation
    c. Dropped film corner
    d. Elongated image

81. Short teeth with blunted roots appear on the film when:
    a. The vertical angulation is excessive.
    b. The vertical angulation is insufficient.
    c. The horizontal angulation is incorrect.

d. There is a cone cut.

82. Blurred images appear on the film when:

   a. There is patient movement
   b. The film is reversed.
   c. There is a double exposure.
   d. The film is creased.

83. When the film is reversed, the image will be:
   a. Elongated
   b. Distorted
   c. Light with herringbone or lower jaw
   d. Blurred

84. The occlusal technique is used to examine:
   a. Interproximal areas
   b. Large areas of the upper or lower jaw
   c. Third molars
   d. For bone loss

85. In children, size ____ film is used in the occlusal examination.
   a. 0
   b. 1
   c. 2
   d. 4

86. When the occlusal technique is used, a ____ to stabilize the film.
   a. Stabe bite-block is used
   b. Hemostat is used
   c. Patient gently bites on the surface of the film
   d. Bite-wing tab is used

87. For the maxillary topographic occlusal projection, the central ray is directed at ____degrees.
   a. +30
   b. +45
   c. +65
   d. -30

88. When the right-angle technique is used, an occlusal film is exposed directing the central ray at ___degrees to the film.
    a. 20
    b. 45
    c. 65
    d. 90

89. For the mandibular topographic occlusal projection, position the PID so that the central ray is directed at ___degrees toward the center of the film.
    a. +55
    b. -55
    c. +90
    d. -90

90. Green-Sensitive film must be paired with intensifying screens that produce___light.
    a. Yellow
    b. Blue
    c. Red
    d. Green

91. The most common extraoral film is the ___projection.
    a. Lateral cephalometric
    b. Posteroanterior
    c. Waters
    d. Panoramic radiograph

92. Extraoral radiographs may be used in conjunction with intraoral films. The images seen on extraoral film are not as defined or sharp as the images seen on an intraoral radiograph.
    a. Both statements are true.
    b. Both statements are false.
    c. The first statement is true; The second statement is false.
    d. The first statement is false; the second statement is false.

93. Which of the following is the fastest recommended screen and screen film combination?
    a. Calcium tungstate screen with blue light
    b. Calcium tungstate screen with green light
    c. Rare earth screen with blue light
    d. Rare earth screen with green light

94. To compensate for the strips found in the grid, ___must be used to expose a film.
    a. Increased kilovoltage
    b. Increased milliamperage
    c. Increased exposure time
    d. Decreased exposure time

95. Radiographs are intended to be placed in a film holder in:
    a. The order in which they are exposed
    b. The order in which they were processed
    c. Anatomic order
    d. The order prescribed by the ADA nomenclature

96. In dental radiography, film mounting is the placement of radiographs:
    a. On a viewbox
    b. In a supporting structure or holder
    c. In the patient's mouth
    d. In the processor

97. Which of the following structures appears as a radiolucency on panoramic radiographs?
    a. Lateral pterygoid plate
    b. Medial pterygoid plate
    c. Pterygomaxillary fissure
    d. Coronoid process

98. On a panoramic radiograph the coronoid notch appears as a ___to the coronoid process.
    a. Concavity located mesial
    b. Concavity located distal
    c. Convexity located mesial

d. Convexity located distal

99. On a panoramic radiograph the ear is viewed superimposed over the:
    a. Anterior teeth
    b. Styloid process
    c. Incisive foramen
    d. Mandibular canal

100. In the dental setting, interpretation refers to an explanation of what is viewed on a radiograph, whereas the term diagnosis refers to the identification of disease by examination or analysis.
    a. Both statements are true.
    b. Both statements are false.
    c. The first statement is true; the second statement is false.
    d. The first statement is false; the second statement is true.

Answer Sheet

1. _____
2. _____
3. _____
4. _____
5. _____
6. _____
7. _____
8. _____
9. _____
10. _____
11. _____
12. _____
13. _____
14. _____
15. _____
16. _____
17. _____
18. _____
19. _____
20. _____
21. _____
22. _____
23. _____
24. _____
25. _____
26. _____
27. _____
28. _____
29. _____
30. _____
31. _____
32. _____
33. _____
34. _____
35. _____
36. _____
37. _____
38. _____
39. _____
40. _____
41. _____
42. _____
43. _____
44. _____
45. _____
46. _____
47. _____
48. _____
49. _____
50. _____
51. _____
52. _____
53. _____
54. _____
55. _____
56. _____
57. _____
58. _____
59. _____
60. _____
61. _____
62. _____
63. _____
64. _____
65. _____
66. _____
67. _____
68. _____
69. _____
70. _____
71. _____
72. _____
73. _____
74. _____
75. _____
76. _____
77. _____
78. _____
79. _____
80. _____
81. _____
82. _____
83. _____
84. _____
85. _____
86. _____
87. _____
88. _____
89. _____
90. _____
91. _____
92. _____
93. _____
94. _____
95. _____
96. _____
97. _____
98. _____
99. _____
100. _____

Answer Sheet

1. _____
2. _____
3. _____
4. _____
5. _____
6. _____
7. _____
8. _____
9. _____
10. _____
11. _____
12. _____
13. _____
14. _____
15. _____
16. _____
17. _____
18. _____
19. _____
20. _____
21. _____
22. _____
23. _____
24. _____
25. _____
26. _____
27. _____
28. _____
29. _____
30. _____
31. _____
32. _____
33. _____
34. _____
35. _____
36. _____
37. _____
38. _____
39. _____
40. _____
41. _____
42. _____
43. _____
44. _____
45. _____
46. _____
47. _____
48. _____
49. _____
50. _____
51. _____
52. _____
53. _____
54. _____
55. _____
56. _____
57. _____
58. _____
59. _____
60. _____
61. _____
62. _____
63. _____
64. _____
65. _____
66. _____
67. _____
68. _____
69. _____
70. _____
71. _____
72. _____
73. _____
74. _____
75. _____
76. _____
77. _____
78. _____
79. _____
80. _____
81. _____
82. _____
83. _____
84. _____
85. _____
86. _____
87. _____
88. _____
89. _____
90. _____
91. _____
92. _____
93. _____
94. _____
95. _____
96. _____
97. _____
98. _____
99. _____
100. _____

Answer Sheet

1. _____
2. _____
3. _____
4. _____
5. _____
6. _____
7. _____
8. _____
9. _____
10. _____
11. _____
12. _____
13. _____
14. _____
15. _____
16. _____
17. _____
18. _____
19. _____
20. _____
21. _____
22. _____
23. _____
24. _____
25. _____
26. _____
27. _____
28. _____
29. _____
30. _____
31. _____
32. _____
33. _____
34. _____
35. _____
36. _____
37. _____
38. _____
39. _____
40. _____
41. _____
42. _____
43. _____
44. _____
45. _____
46. _____
47. _____
48. _____
49. _____
50. _____
51. _____
52. _____
53. _____
54. _____
55. _____
56. _____
57. _____
58. _____
59. _____
60. _____
61. _____
62. _____
63. _____
64. _____
65. _____
66. _____
67. _____
68. _____
69. _____
70. _____
71. _____
72. _____
73. _____
74. _____
75. _____
76. _____
77. _____
78. _____
79. _____
80. _____
81. _____
82. _____
83. _____
84. _____
85. _____
86. _____
87. _____
88. _____
89. _____
90. _____
91. _____
92. _____
93. _____
94. _____
95. _____
96. _____
97. _____
98. _____
99. _____
100. _____

ANSWER KEY

1. B
2. B
3. D
4. C
5. B
6. C
7. D
8. C
9. B
10. B
11. B
12. A
13. D
14. D
15. C
16. C
17. A
18. B
19. B
20. A
21. B
22. D
23. A
24. A
25. B
26. C
27. B
28. C
29. D
30. C
31. B
32. B
33. C
34. D
35. C
36. A
37. D
38. B
39. B
40. A
41. A
42. B
43. A
44. C
45. A
46. D
47. A
48. A
49. C
50. D
51. B
52. B
53. D
54. A
55. A
56. A
57. C
58. A
59. C
60. D
61. B
62. C
63. D
64. A
65. B
66. B
67. B
68. B
69. D
70. A
71. C
72. B
73. C
74. C
75. B
76. B
77. B
78. D
79. A
80. C
81. A
82. A
83. C
84. B
85. C
86. C
87. C
88. D
89. B
90. D
91. D
92. A
93. D
94. C
95. C
96. B
97. C
98. B
99. B
100. A

FREE RESOURCES

WEBSITE CREATED BY AUTHOR OF BOOK TO HELP YOU WITH PLACEMENT OF RADIOGRAPHS AND MORE

https://dentalindexjr.weebly.com/radiology--danb-rhs-lecture.html

HTTPS://DENTALINDEX.WEEBLY.COM FOR ALL DENTAL PROFESSIONALS
HTTPS://DENTALINDEXJR.WEEBLY.COM FOR ALL DENTAL STUDENTS

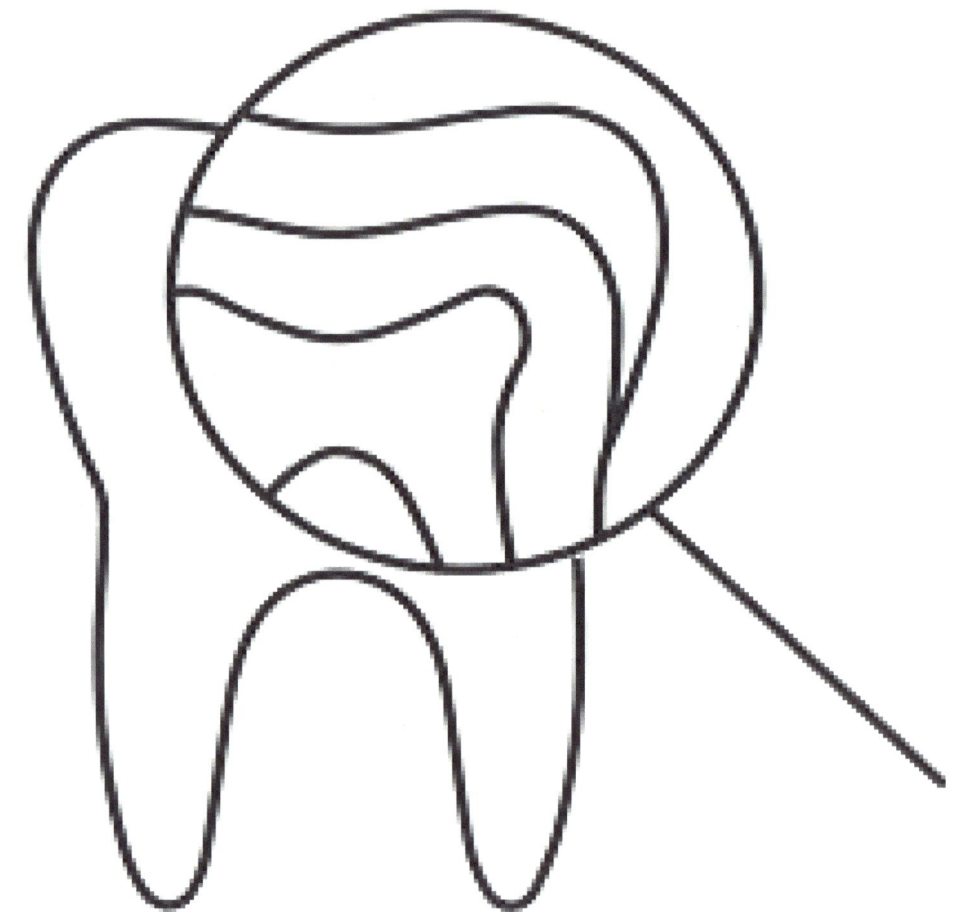

COLOR AND LABEL

FOR ONES YOU GOT WRONG ON TEST MAKE FLASH CARDS UP AND TEAR FROM BOOK! WHEN YOU TYPE OR WRITE IT YOU WILL RECALL IT WHEN NEED TO!

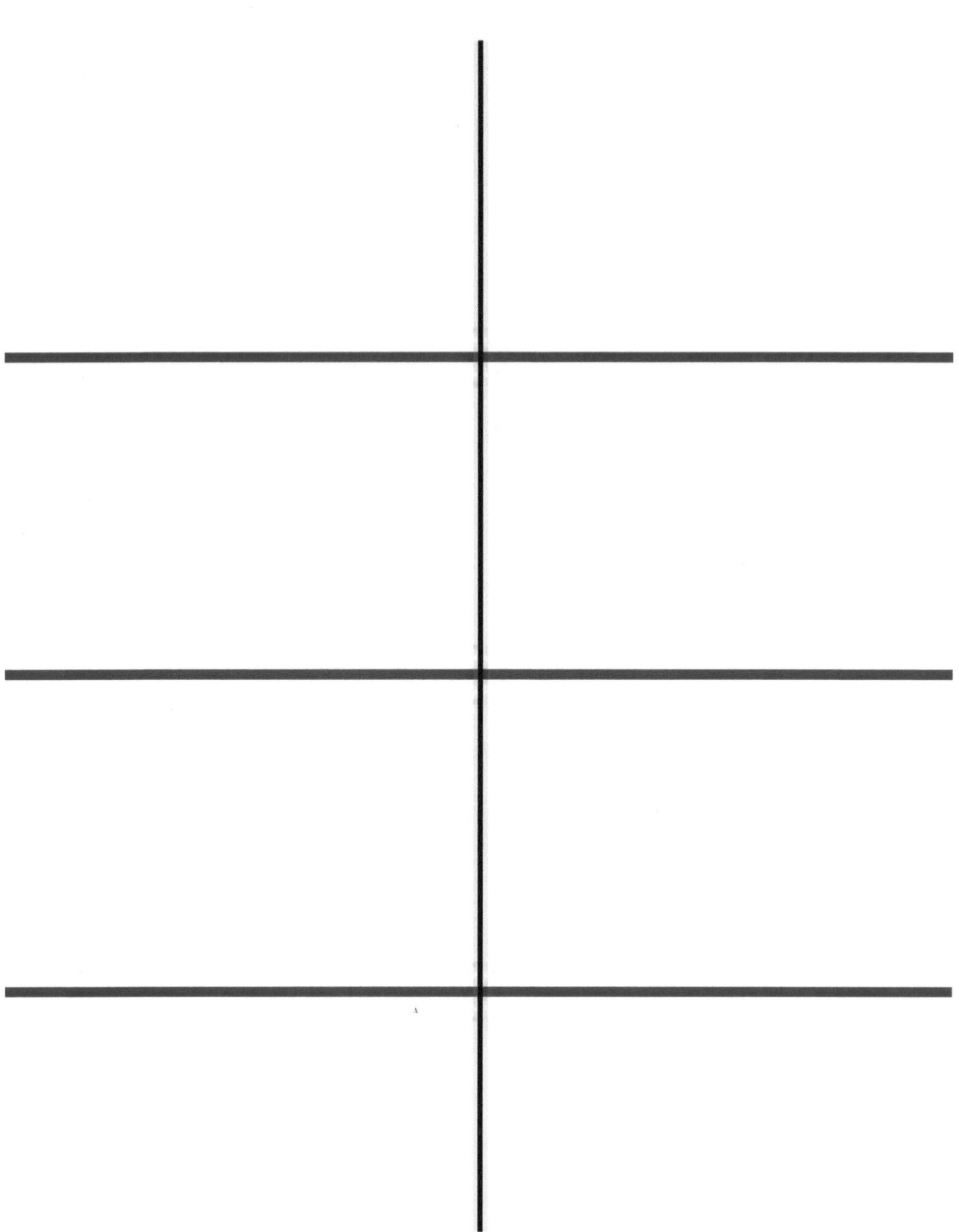

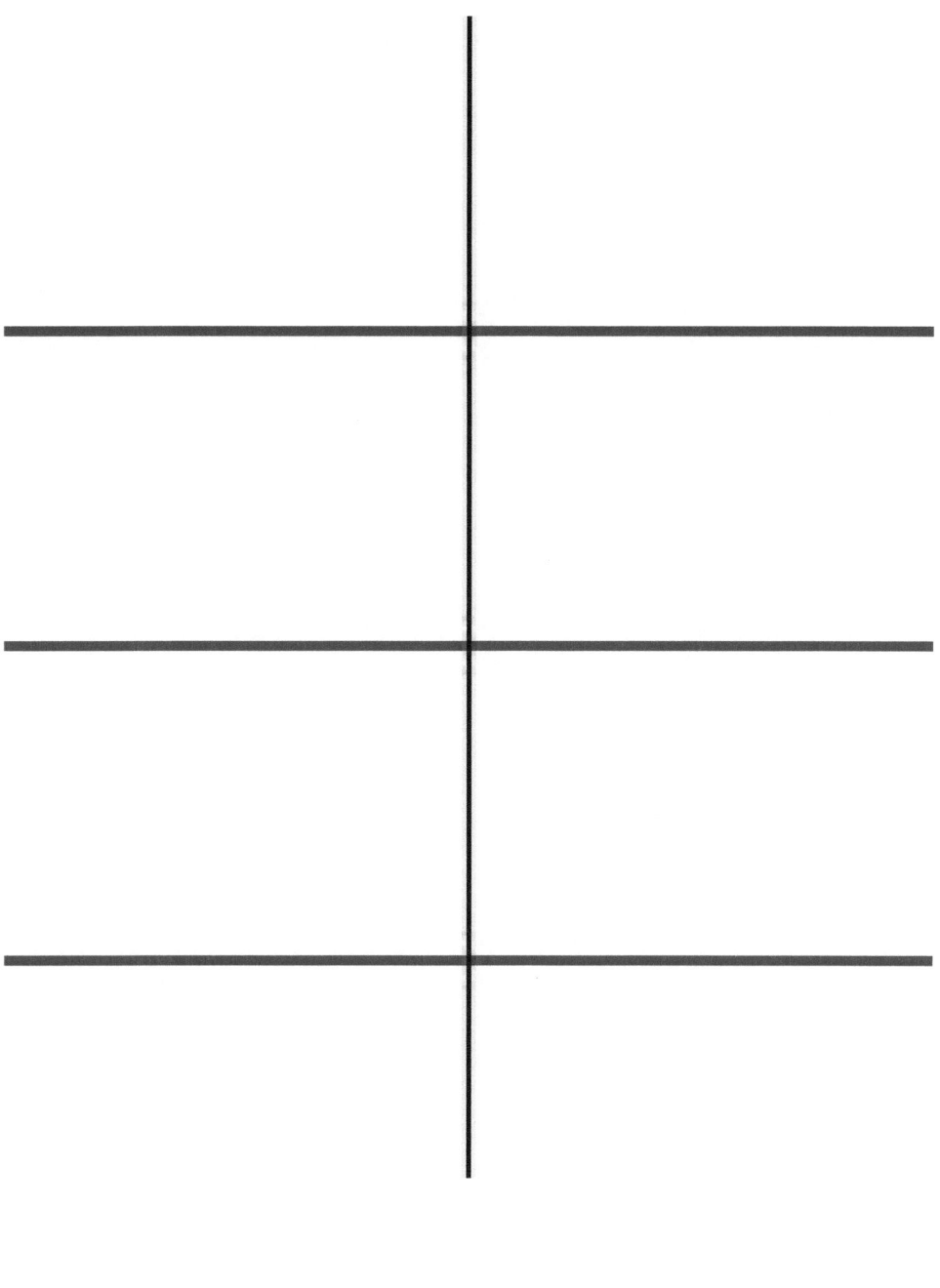

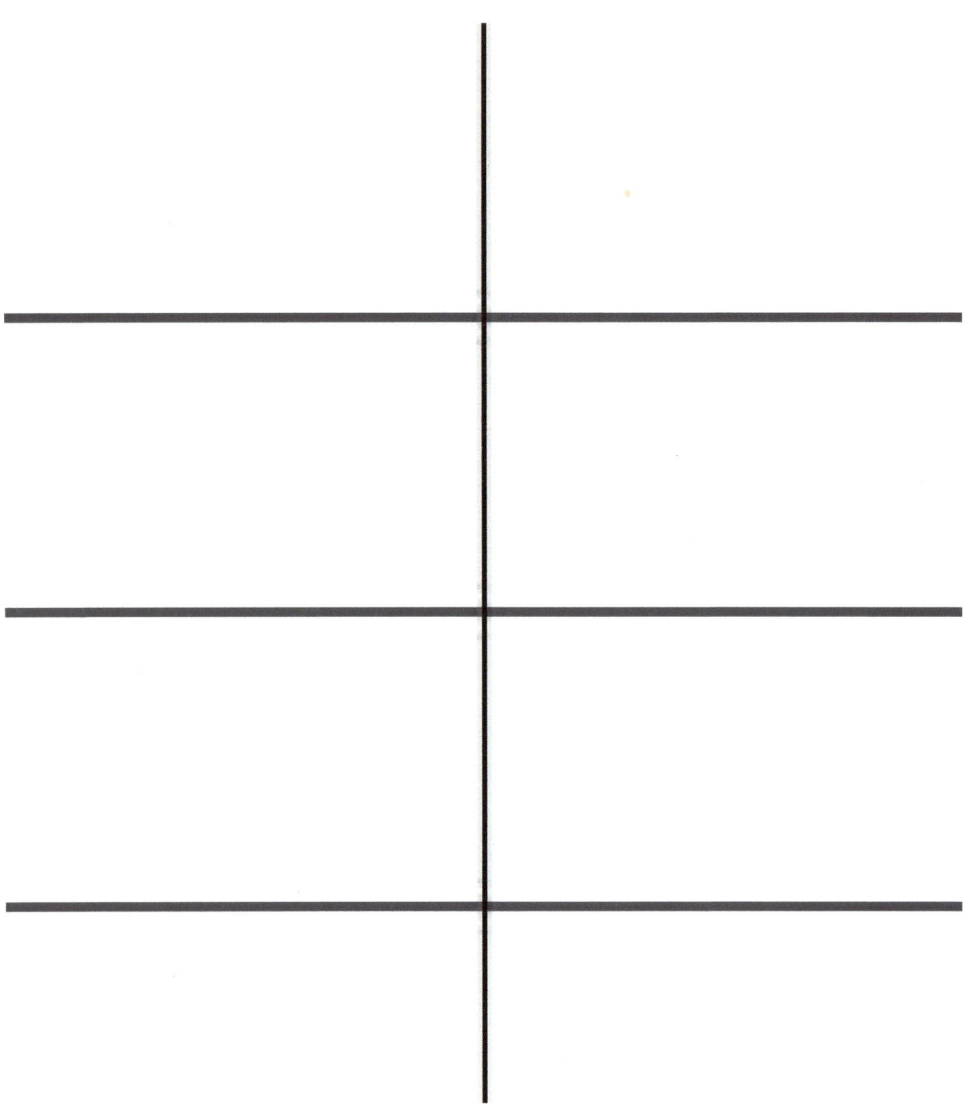

OR MAKE SOME ONLINE FOR FREE!

https://quizlet.com/login

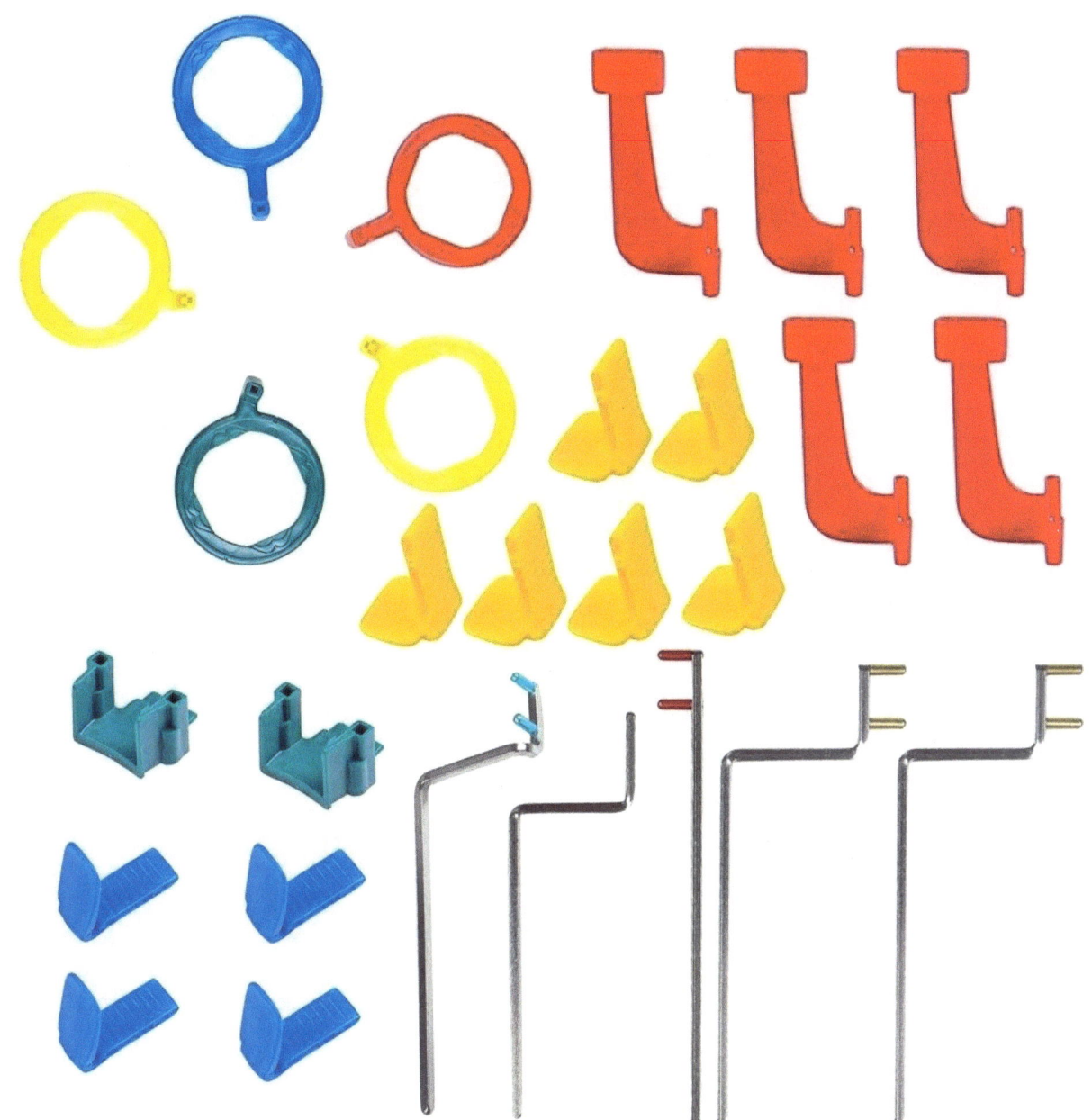

LABEL

BLUE FOR _____

RED _____

YELLOW _____

GREEN _____

HORZONTAL _____

VERTICAL _____

USE DENTAL ASSISTANT TEXTBOOK OR
https://dentalindexjr.weebly.com/radiology--danb-rhs-lecture.html FOR ANSWERS

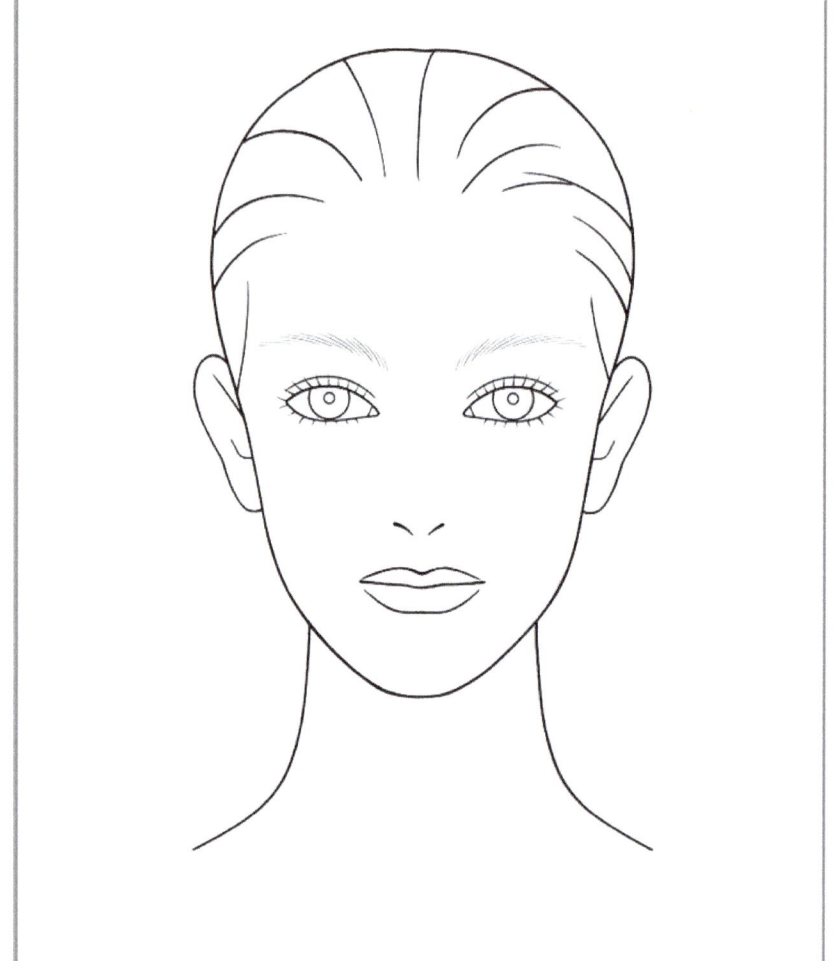

LABEL THE PATIENT ABOVE WITH THE LANDMARKS LISTED BELOW

- Take your finger and touch your nose and follow it straight down over your lip , What teeth are those ? Your Centrals! Use this landmark in placing a Rinn Kit.
- Take your finger and from the inside of your eyebrow and go straight down that takes you to your Lateral & Cuspids
- Take your finger and don't put your finger in your eye lol but right below the pupil follow down that will take you to the Premolars also called Bi-Cuspids.
- Take your finger and outside of the eyebrow go straight down and that is your Molars.
- Take your finger this time and take it to the earlobe and take the other to the inner part of the eyebrow, that's how you line up for premolar Bitewings.

COLOR EACH PART DIFFERENT TO HELP STUDY THE LAYOUT AND YOU WILL NEED TO KNOW AND UNDERSTAND THE LAYOUT OF INSIDE THE TUBEHEAD.

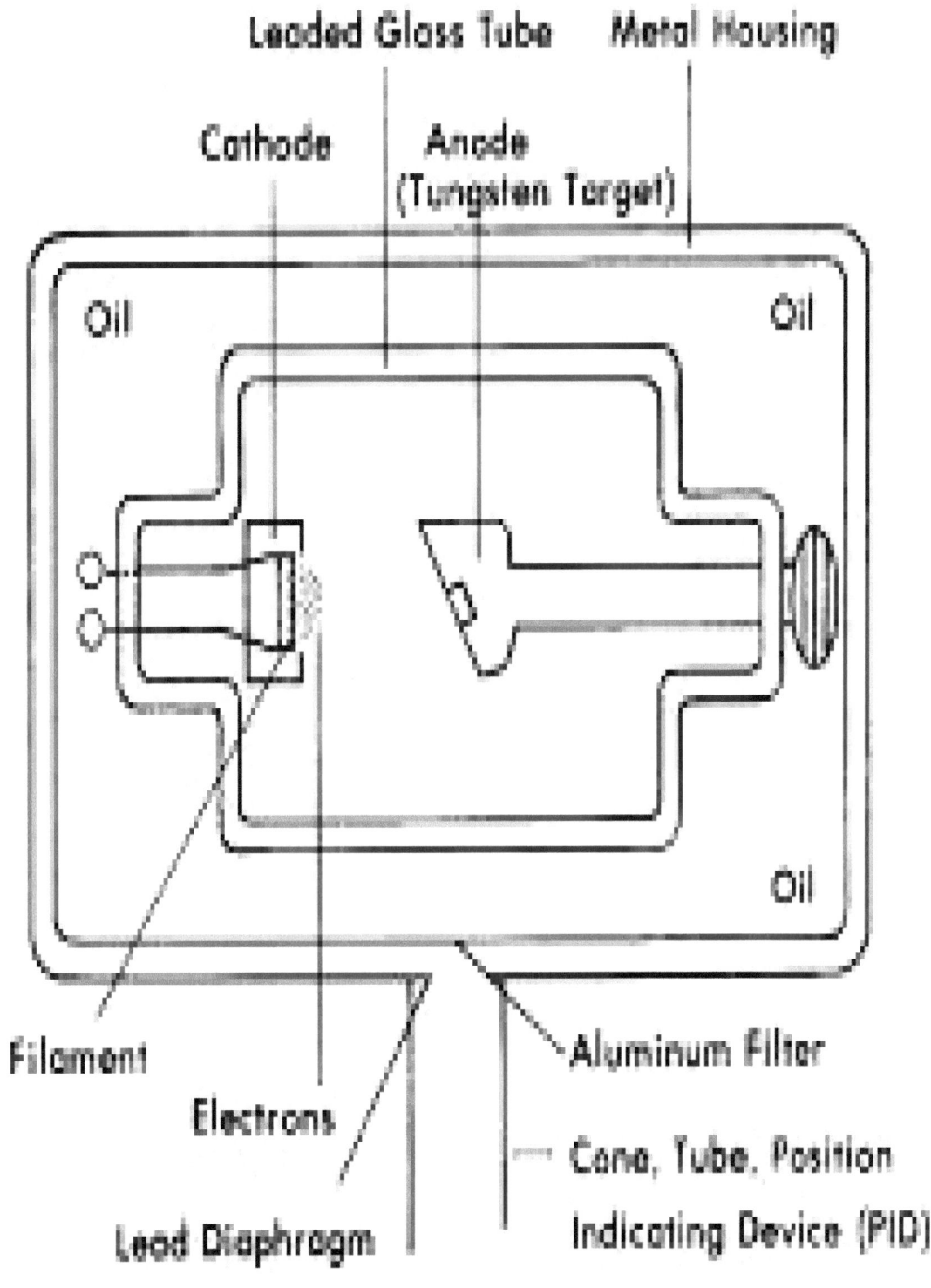

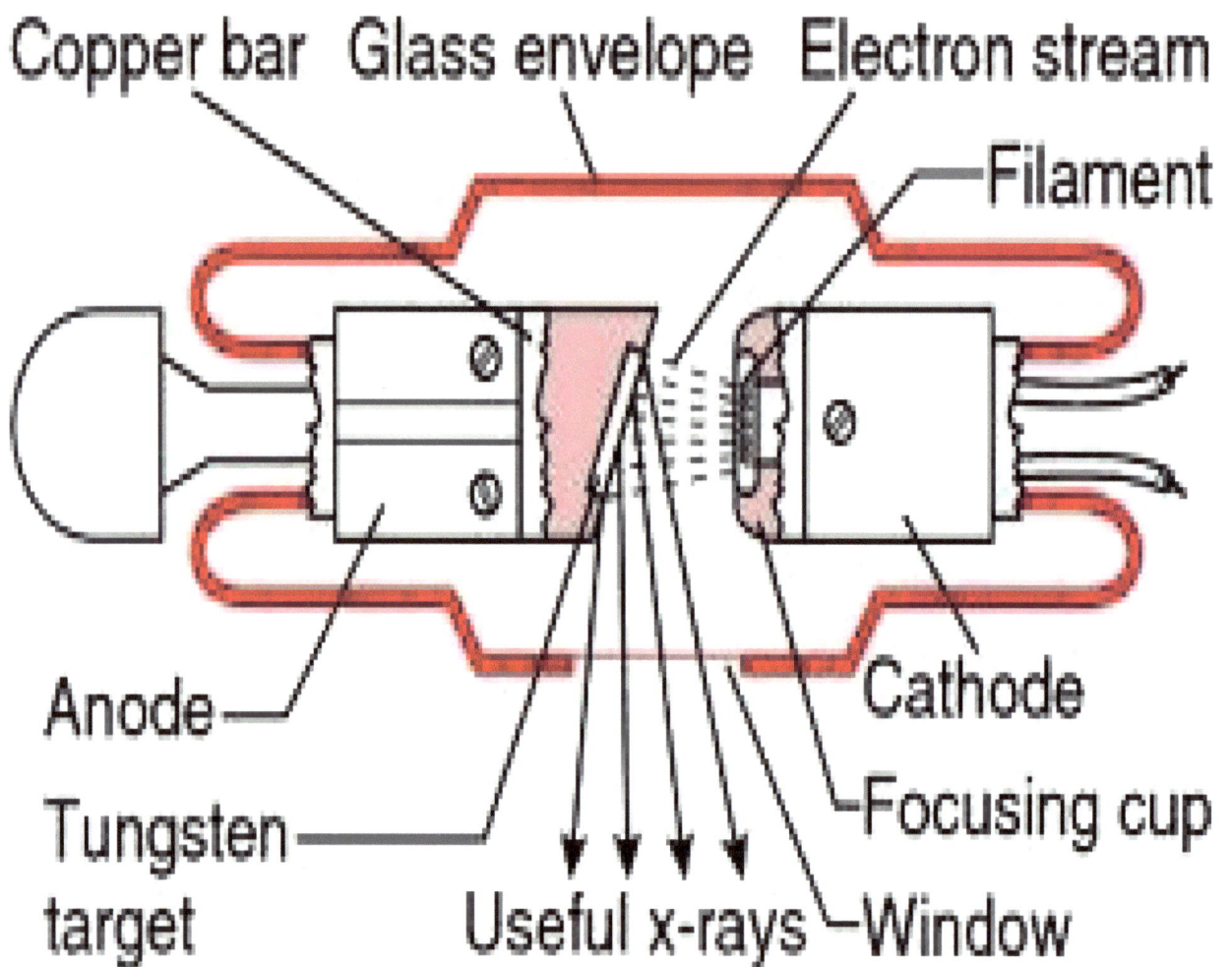

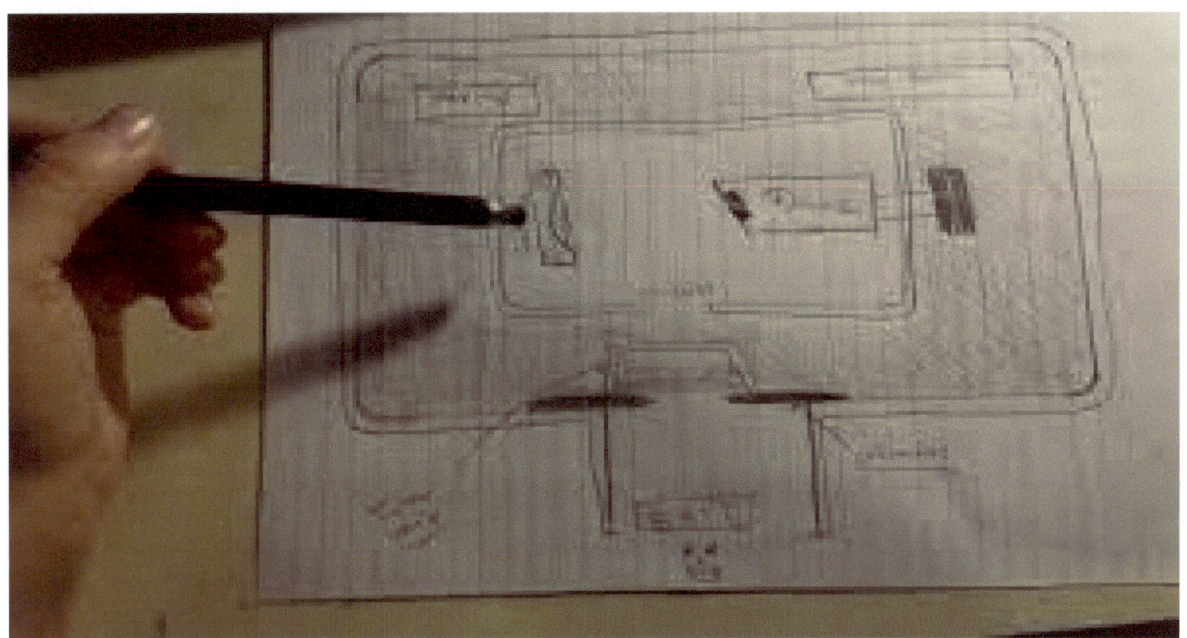

EVEN GRAB A PIECE OF PAPER AND DRAW IT FREE HAND TO HELP YOUR MEMORY RECALL IT WHILE TESTING. YOUR NERVES MIGHT GET THE BEST OF YOU SO RELAX AND JUST HAVE FUN STUDYING BY DRAWING IT. YOU BE GLAD THAT YOU DID. USE SPACE BELOW!

COLOR AND LABEL EVEN WRITE IN THE DEGREES (+) OR (-)

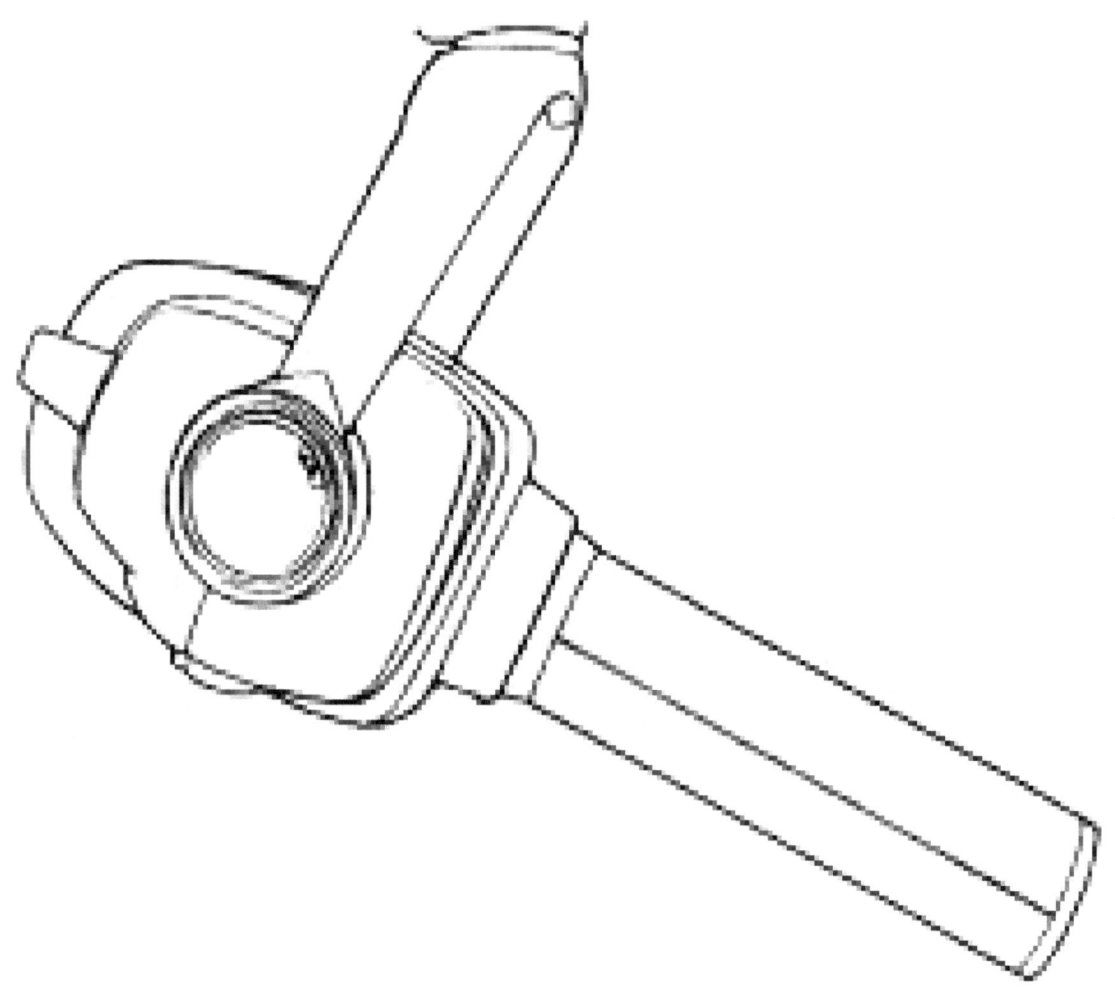

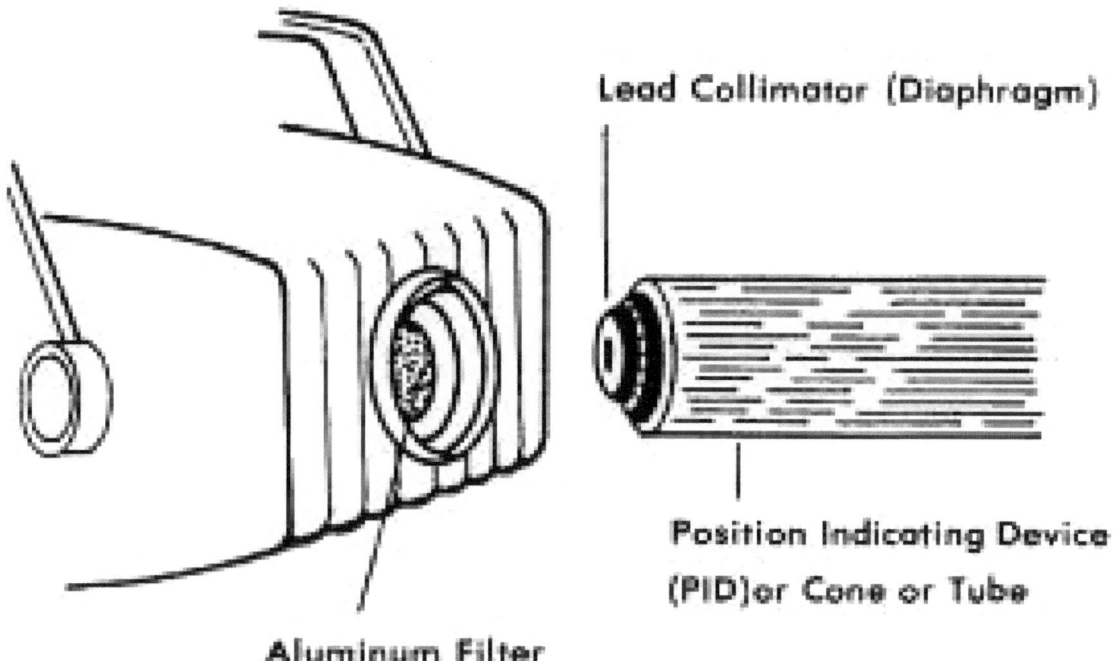

Lead Collimator (Diaphragm)

Position Indicating Device (PID) or Cone or Tube

Aluminum Filter

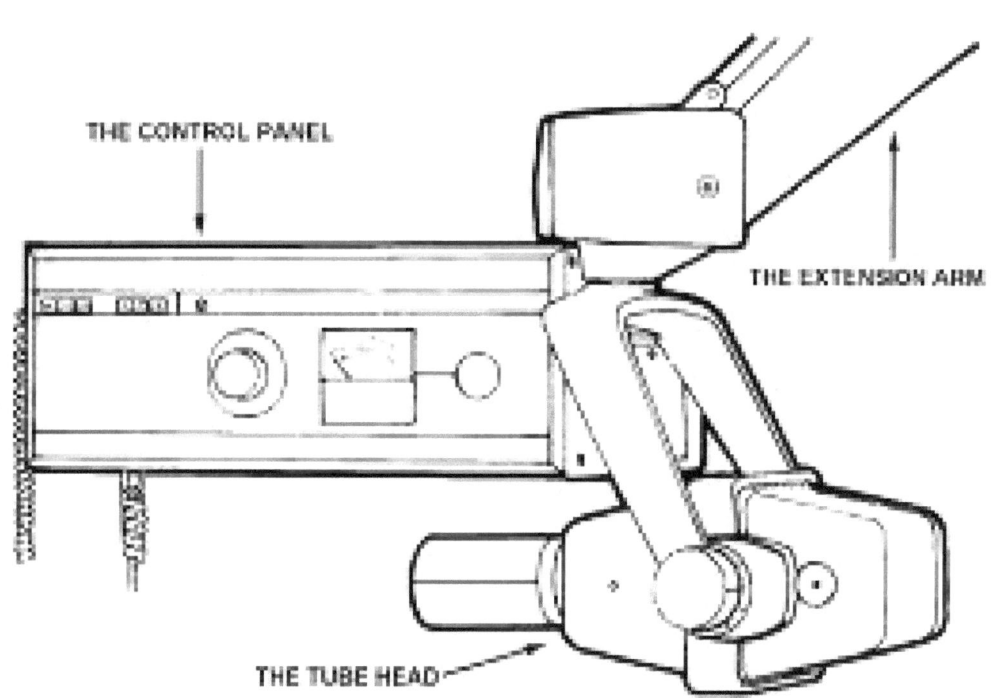

THE CONTROL PANEL

THE EXTENSION ARM

THE TUBE HEAD

KNOW YOUR PROCEDURE CODES FOR X-RAYS TO SAVE TIME NOTICE THE BITEWINGS FOR EXAMPLE ARE 0272 FOR 2 AND FOR 4 0274

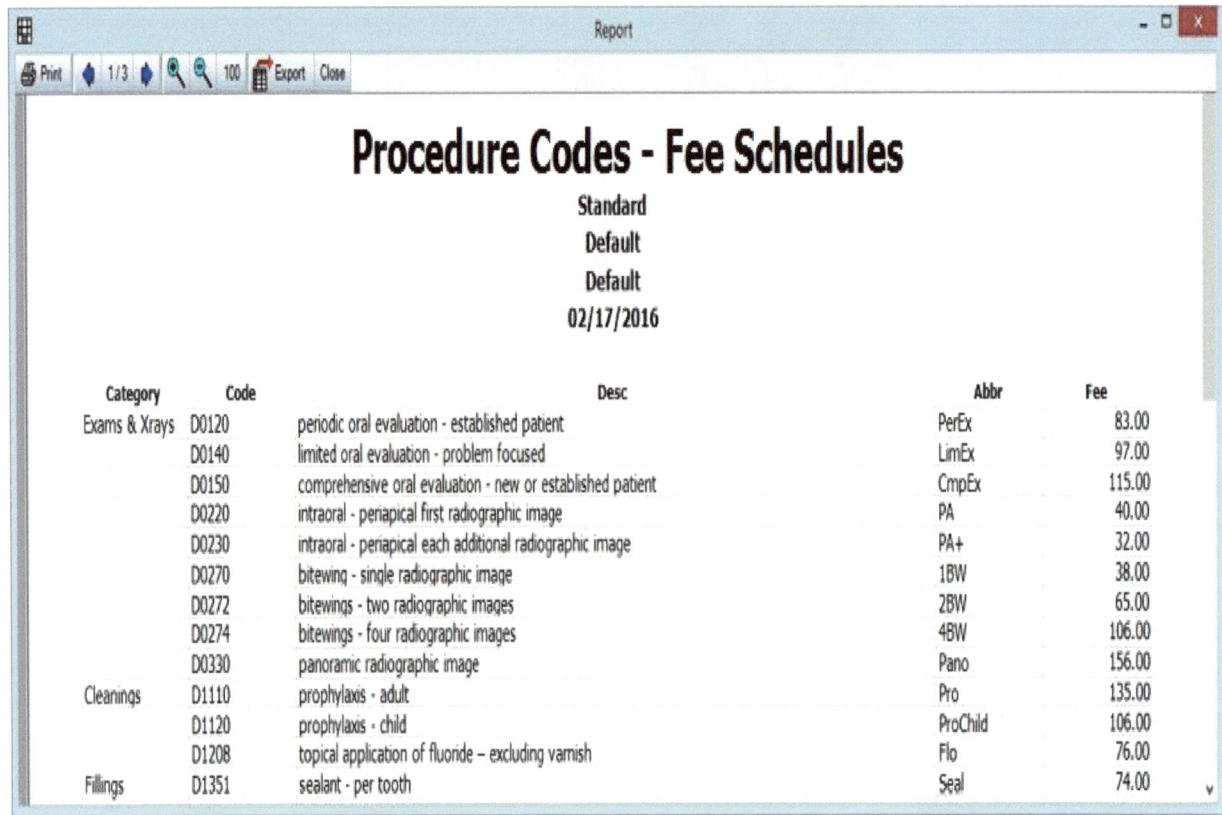

MAKE A CHEAT SHEET ON A POSTED NOTE IN KEEP INSIDE TREATMENT CABINET OR SAVE HTTPS://DENTALINDEXJR.WEEBLY.COM ON YOUR HOME SCREEN OF PHONE TO CLICK AND LOOK!

CP12H6V

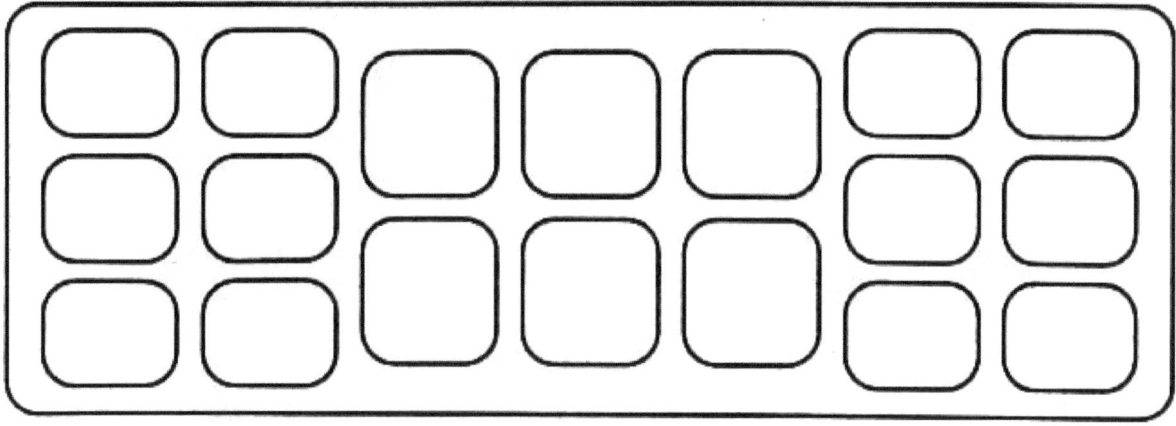

FMX- 18 windows

DRAW THE TEETH IN THE MOUNT WITH A PENCIL IF YOU CAN DRAW IT YOU WILL ETCH IT INTO YOUR MEMORY. PLUS A FUN WAY TO LEARN
USE ONE BELOW FOR COMPARISON!

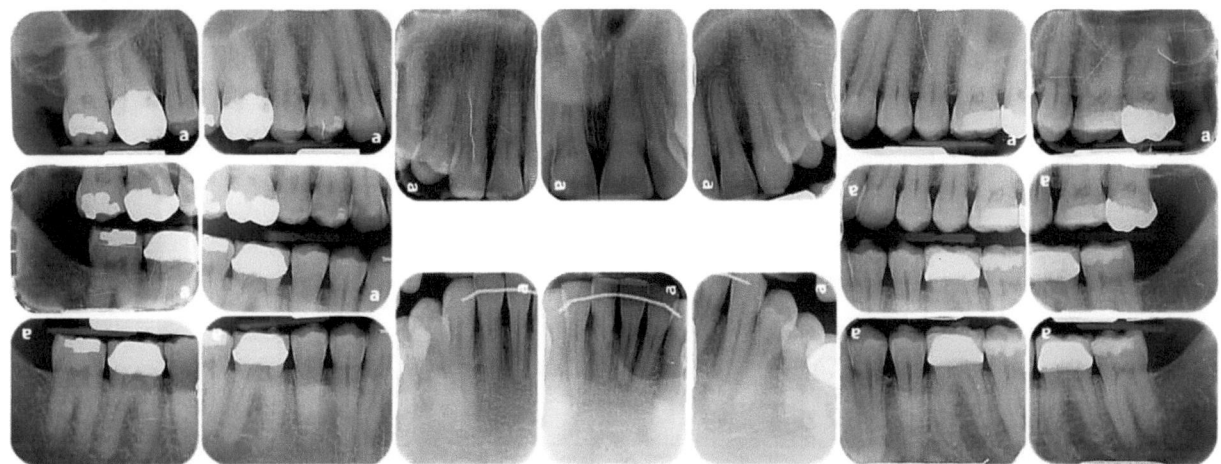

OR CUT OUT OF BOOK AND LEARN HOW TO MOUNT THEM IN RIGHT ORDER PLACING THEM ON THE MOUNT IN ORDER AS IN MOUTH BEFORE CUTTING AND MIXING UP TAKE PHOTO WITH PHONE TO REMIND YOU HOW IT WAS IN ORDER.

IF KINDLE BOOK SCREEN SHOT AND PRINT OUT OR USE NOTE PEN FOR PHONE IF ABLE.

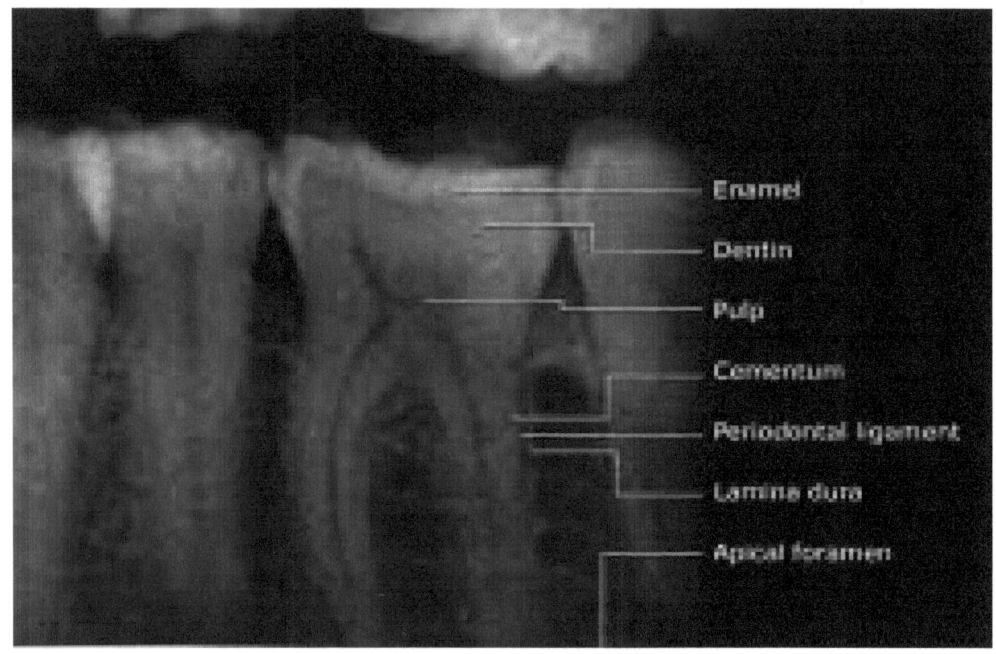

USE TO PHOTO TO LABEL PHOTO BELOW

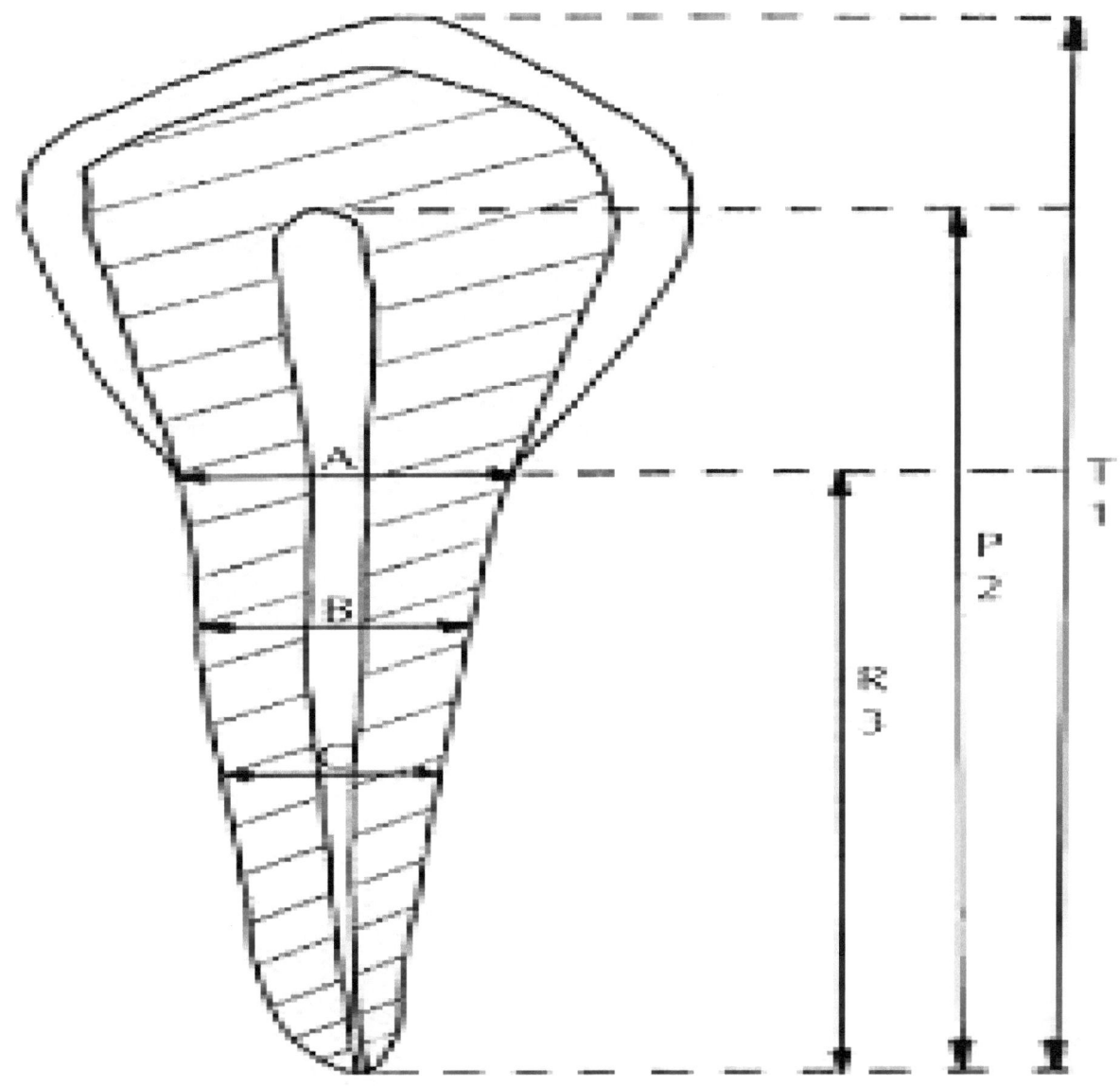

KNOW THE TOOTH YOU ARE X-RAYING THE LAYERS OF EACH TOOTH ARE ALL THE SAME. KNOW WHICH SURFACES OR MATERIALS ARE MORE RADIOLUCENT OR RADIOPAQUE FOR EXAM COLOR IN AND LABEL!

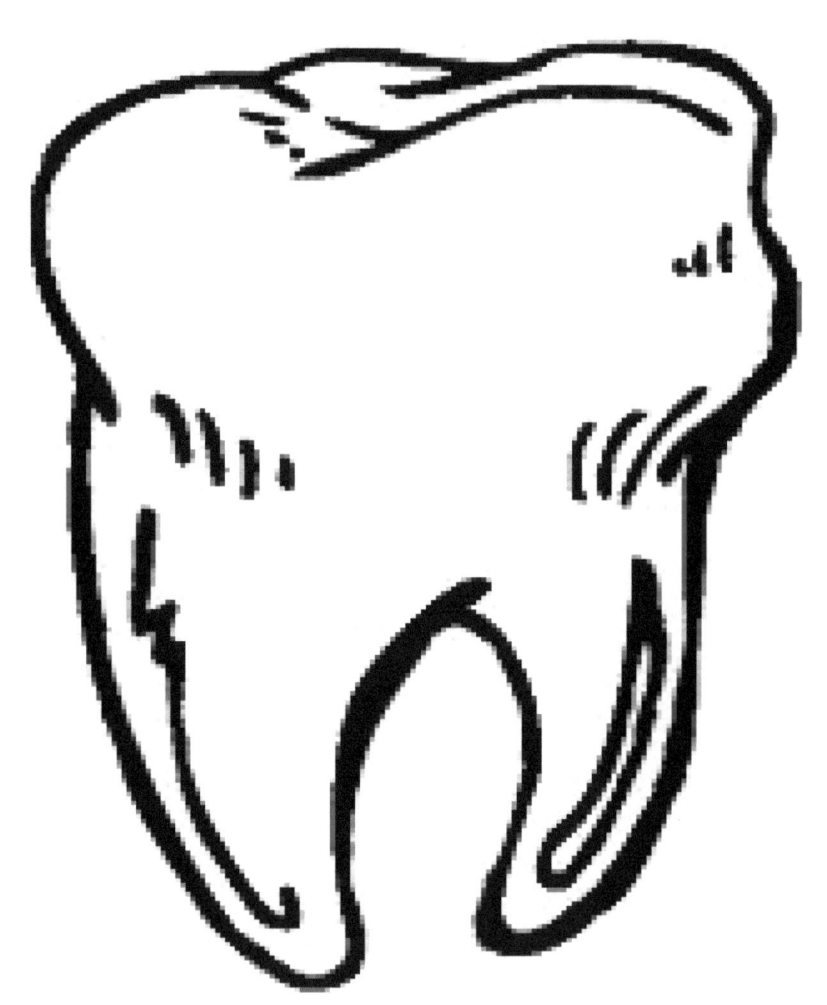

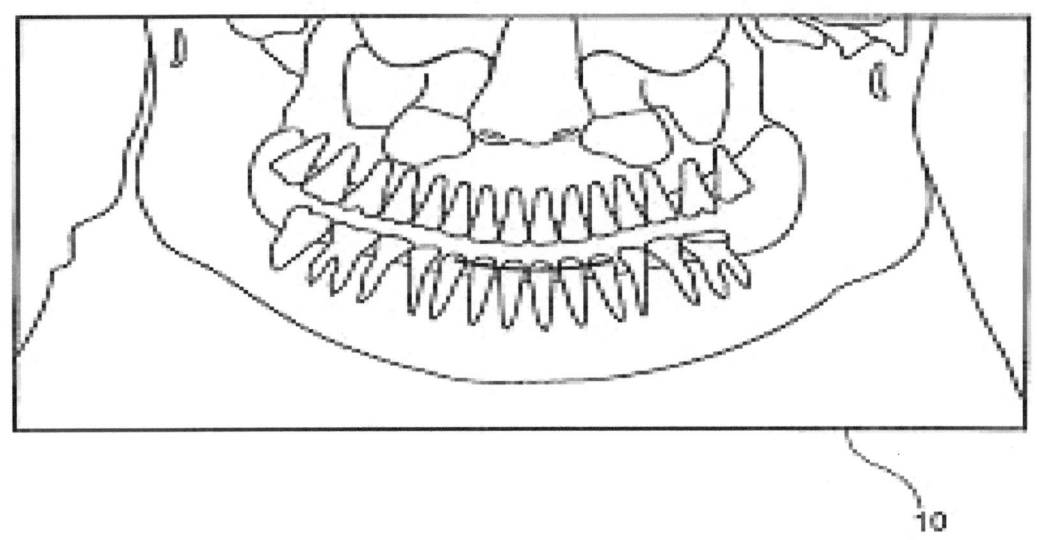

COLOR AND LABEL INCASE ON TEST YOUR ASKED LANDMARK

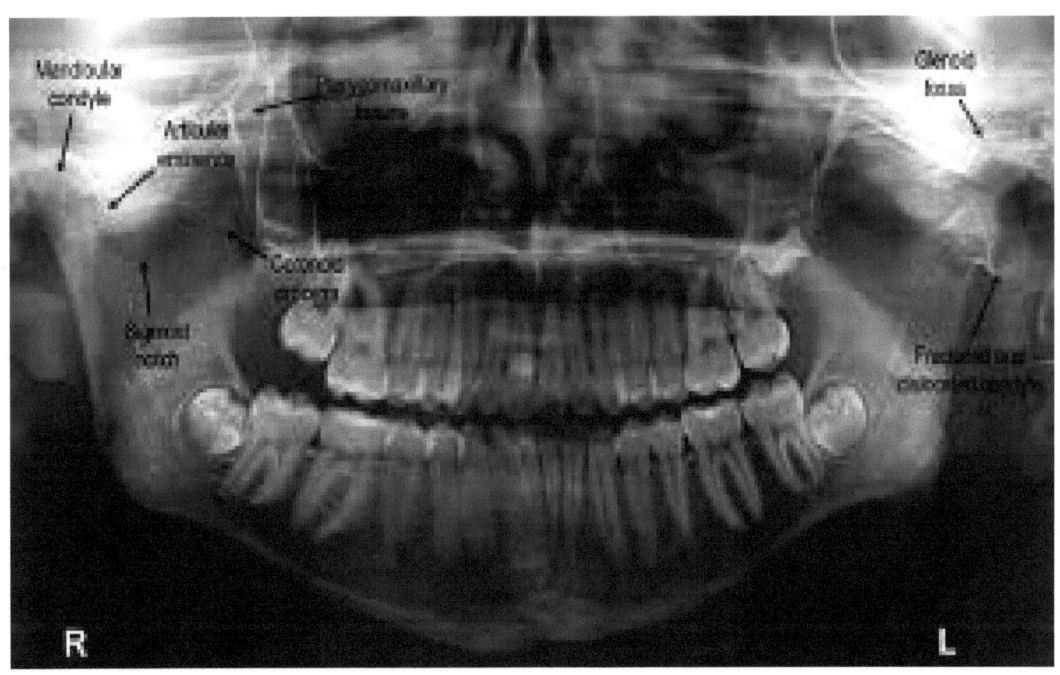

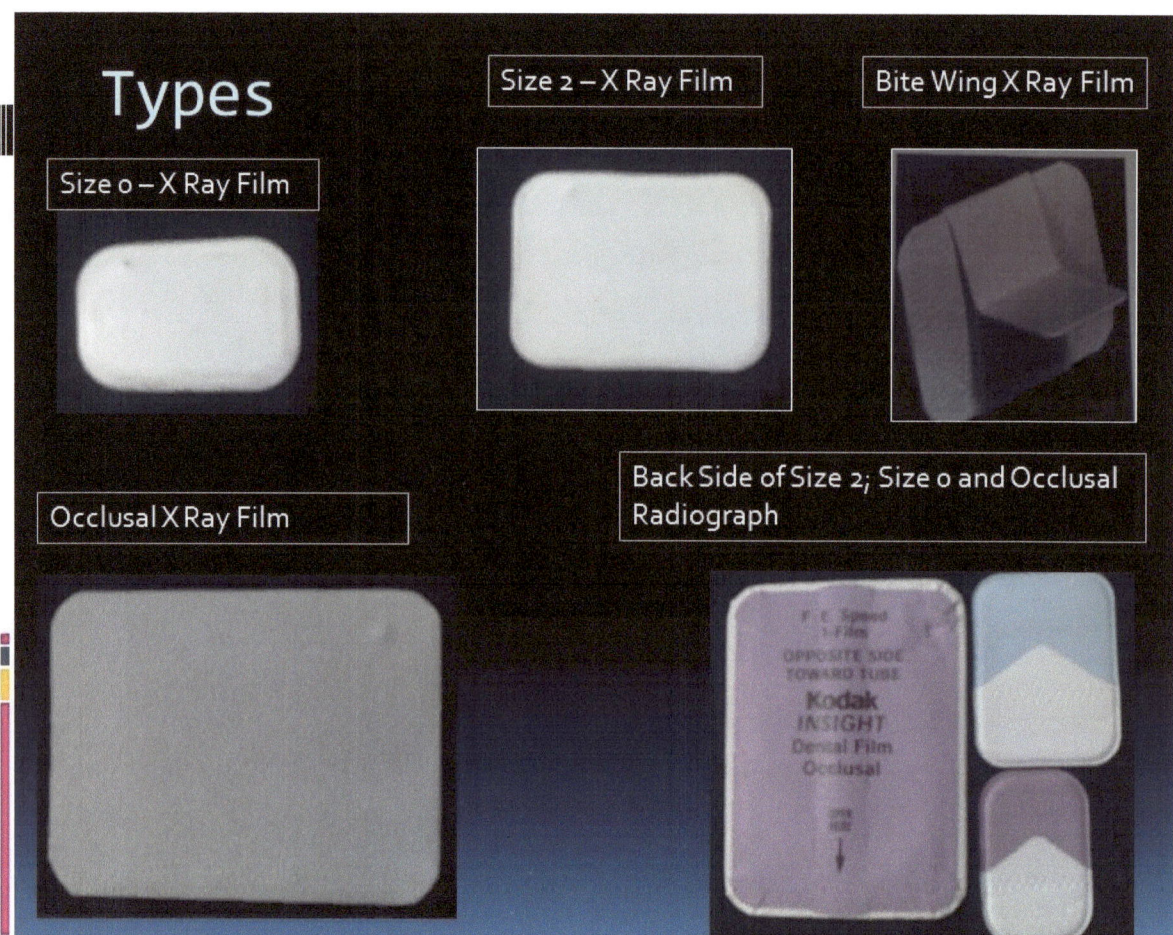

REMEMBER YOU CAN DO THIS! STUDY STUDY STUDY!

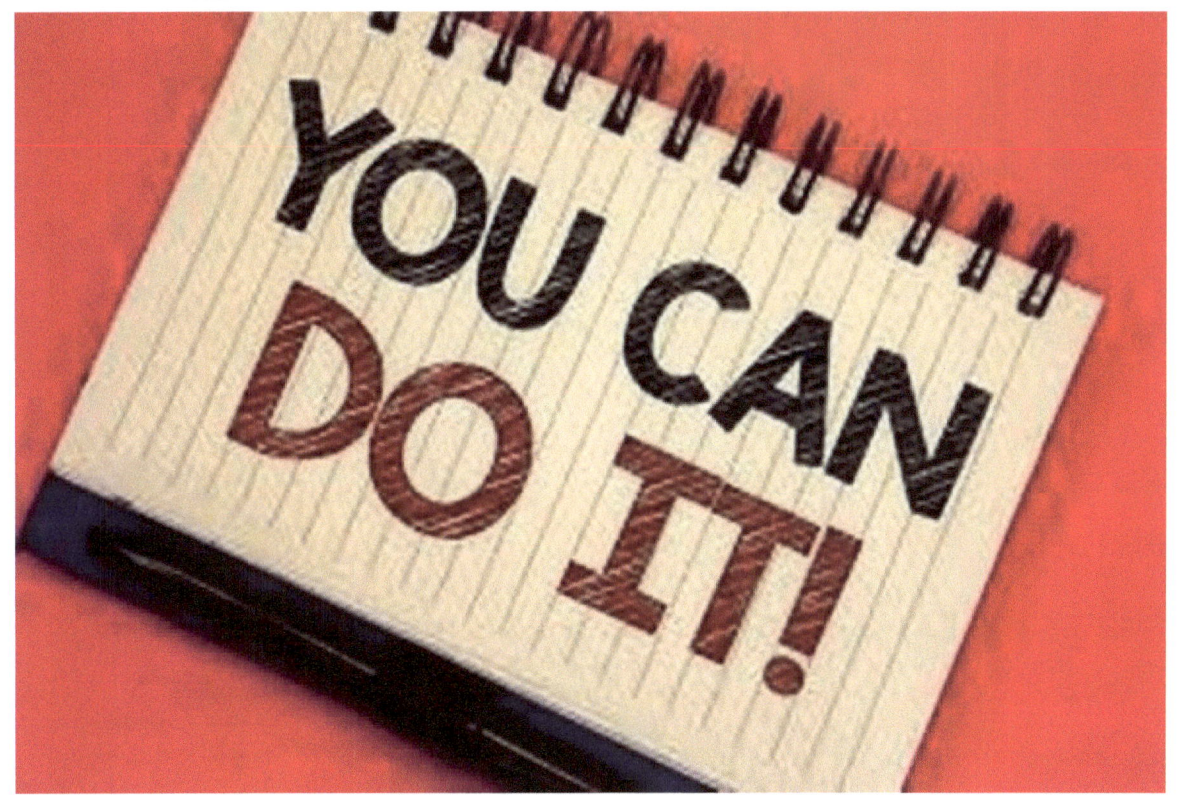

PLACES TO SIGN UP TO TAKE EXAM
DANB
https://www.danb.org/Become-Certified/Exams-and-Certifications/RHS-Exam.aspx
DENT ED ONLINE
https://www.dent-ed-online.com/pages/homepage.php?course=radiology&course_type=ondemand

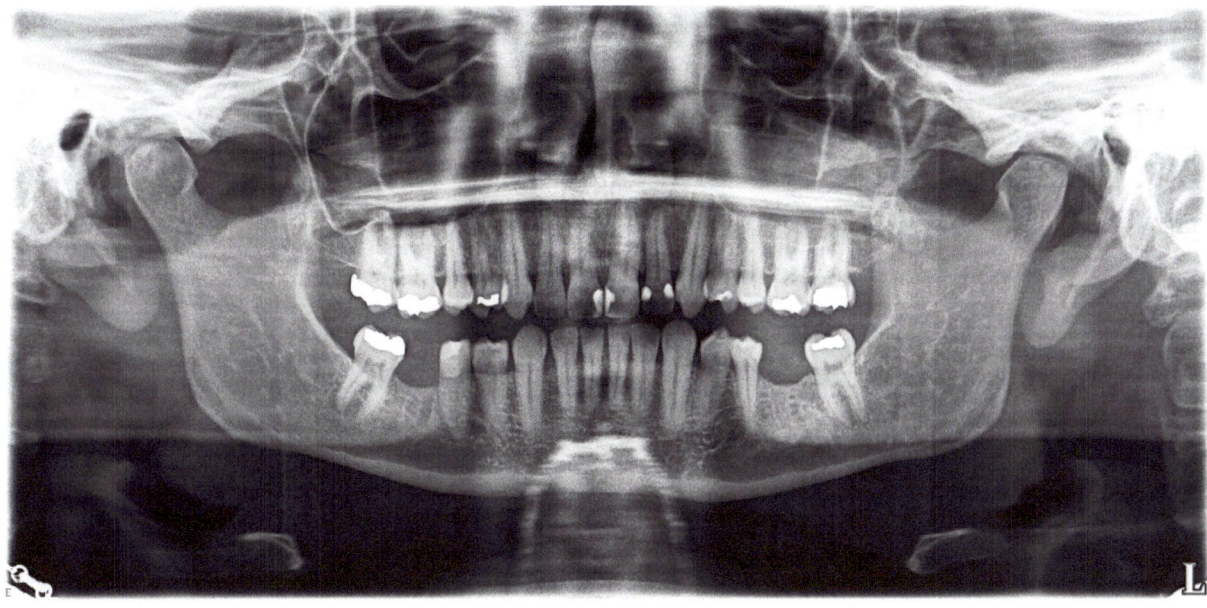

SPECIAL DATES!

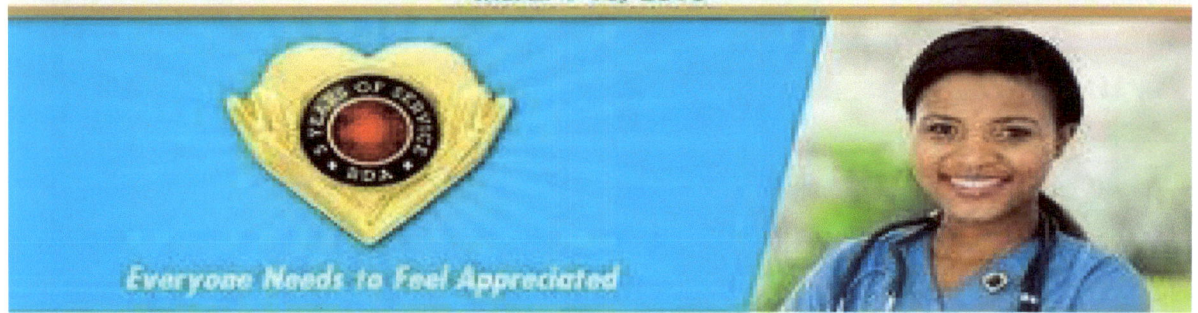

OTHER BOOKS BY AUTHOR THERESA BIGGS RDA, CDA-DENTAL INSTRUCTOR

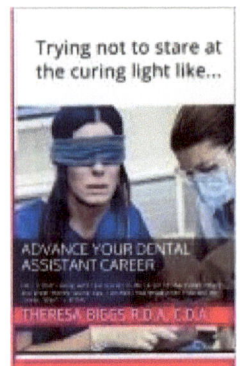 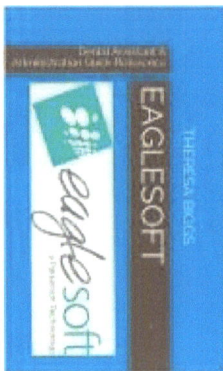 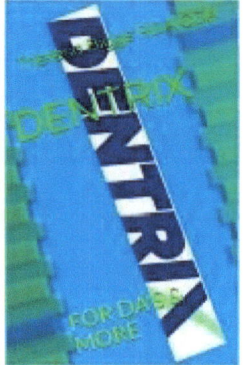 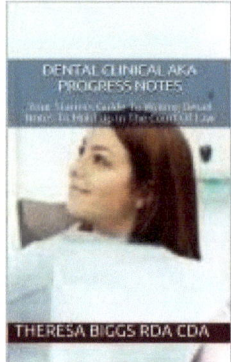 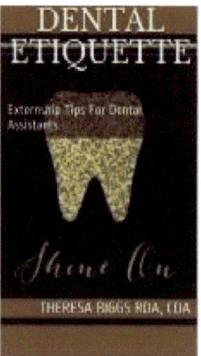

Also In Spanish
Radiology video
https://www.youtube.com/watch?v=jrVSAds9Tgg&list=PLflGPioUGGVogiKewUjFGFOxBExBwHLwh
Website
https://dentalindexjr.weebly.com/radiology--danb-rhs-lecture.html

CDA Review
https://dentalindexjr.weebly.com/danb-cda-review.html

Good Luck and Rest Well The Night Before!

www.ingramcontent.com/pod-product-compliance
Lightning Source LLC
Chambersburg PA
CBHW040411220526
45473CB00004B/1207